Ashley Fitzgerald

SOMATIC THERAPY FOR CANCER

Mind-Body Approaches to Conquering Cancer

Published by UNITEXTO

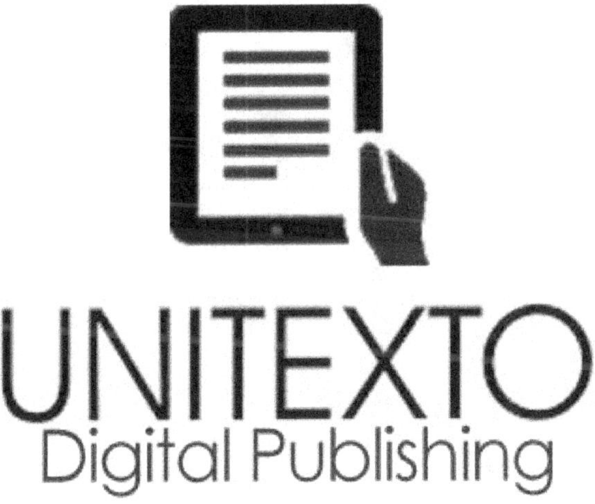

TABLE OF CONTENTS

Why this book?

About the Author

Chapter 1: Understanding Cancer and Its Impacts
- Introduction to cancer: types, causes, and prevalence.
- Physical and emotional impacts of cancer.
- Overview of traditional and alternative cancer treatments.

Chapter 2: Introduction to Somatic Therapy
- Definition and history of somatic therapy.
- Principles and philosophies behind somatic therapy.
- How somatic therapy differs from other therapeutic approaches.

Chapter 3: Somatic Therapy and Cancer Prevention
- Role of somatic therapy in cancer prevention.
- Techniques and exercises for enhancing body awareness.
- Lifestyle changes and habits to reduce cancer risk.

Chapter 4: Somatic Therapy During Cancer Treatment
- How somatic therapy can complement traditional cancer treatments.
- Techniques to manage pain, stress, and side effects of cancer treatments.
- Case studies and patient experiences.

Chapter 5: Body Awareness and Mindfulness
- Deepening body awareness through mindfulness practices.
- Mind-body connection and its significance in cancer treatment.
- Guided exercises for mindfulness and relaxation.

Chapter 6: Emotional Healing and Trauma Release
- Addressing emotional trauma associated with cancer.
- Techniques for emotional release and healing.
- Importance of psychological support during cancer treatment.

Chapter 7: Physical Exercises and Movement Therapy
- Role of physical activity in cancer recovery and prevention.
- Specific somatic exercises and movement therapies.
- Tailoring exercises to individual needs and limitations.

Chapter 8: Nutrition and Lifestyle in Somatic Therapy
- Impact of diet and nutrition on cancer and recovery.
- Somatic approach to eating and food choices.
- Integrating healthy lifestyle choices for holistic healing.

Chapter 9: Building a Supportive Community
- The importance of community and social support.
- Creating and participating in support groups.
- Family, friends, and caregiver roles in somatic therapy.

Chapter 10: Continuing the Journey
- Long-term strategies for maintaining health and preventing recurrence.
- Personal stories of transformation and healing.
- Resources and guidance for further exploration in somatic therapy.

Chapter 11. Case studies

Chapter 12. Weekly activities schedule
-Exercises plan
-Food plan

Chapter 13. References

-Book list
-Academic Open Access Journals
-Searching key words

Why this book

Embracing a New Era in Cancer Treatment

In the world of medical science, a paradigm shift is taking place, one that recognizes the powerful interplay between the mind and body in healing. "Somatic Therapy for Cancer" is at the forefront of this shift, offering a groundbreaking approach to cancer treatment and recovery.

This book is more than just a guide; it is a beacon of hope, illuminating a path that combines the rigor of traditional medicine with the transformative potential of mind-body practices.

Why this book, you may ask? The answer lies in its core philosophy - the belief in the body's inherent ability to heal, supported and amplified by mental and emotional well-being.

In a landscape where cancer treatment often focuses solely on physical symptoms, "Somatic Therapy for Cancer" introduces an integrative approach. It emphasizes the role of somatic therapies in empowering individuals to take an active role in their healing process, harnessing the body's healing power beyond the confines of conventional treatment.

This book is tailored for those touched by cancer – whether you are battling the disease, a caregiver, or a healthcare professional seeking to broaden your treatment modalities.

Its pages are filled with insights into how somatic practices can complement traditional treatments, aiding in symptom management, reducing the side effects of chemotherapy and radiation, and improving overall quality of life.

At its heart, "Somatic Therapy for Cancer" is a testament to the resilience of the human spirit and the body's remarkable capacity for recovery. It blends scientific research with practical advice, providing a holistic roadmap to not just surviving but thriving during and after cancer. The journey through cancer can be daunting, but with this book as your companion, you are not alone. Embrace this new era in cancer treatment, where the mind and body work in concert to conquer one of life's greatest challenges.

Here are compelling reasons to buy and read "Somatic Therapy for Cancer":

1. **Innovative Approach to Cancer Care:**
    This book introduces a pioneering perspective on treating cancer, focusing on somatic therapies that integrate mind and body practices. It offers new insights and techniques that go beyond traditional medical treatments, providing a holistic approach to healing.

2. **Evidence-Based Strategies:**
    "Somatic Therapy for Cancer" is grounded in scientific research and clinical studies. It presents evidence-based strategies that have shown effectiveness in improving the well-being of cancer patients, making it a valuable resource for those seeking reliable and proven methods for cancer care.

3. **Empowerment in the Healing Journey:**
    The book empowers readers by offering tools and practices that they can actively use in their healing process. It emphasizes the role of the individual in their own treatment and recovery, fostering a sense of control and involvement in their health journey.

4. **Support for Mental and Emotional Health:**
    Cancer treatment is often focused on physical health,
    but this book acknowledges and addresses the mental
    and emotional challenges that come with a cancer
    diagnosis. It provides guidance on managing stress,
    anxiety, and other emotional aspects of dealing with
    cancer.

5. **Practical Advice and Techniques:**
    The book is not only theoretical but also highly
    practical. It includes specific techniques, exercises, and
    practices that readers can incorporate into their daily
    lives. This practical advice makes it a useful tool for
    both cancer patients and caregivers, offering tangible
    ways to enhance quality of life during and after
    treatment.

Ashley Fitzgerald

About the Author:

From a tender age, I, Ashley Fitzgerald, was acutely attuned to the nuances of health and personal well-being. These early inklings of self-awareness were not just passing contemplations but the seeds of a lifelong journey towards self-improvement and healing. As the chapters of life unfolded, I embraced my calling with fervor, transforming my youthful concerns into a robust career that spans two decades.

Today, I stand before you not merely as a practitioner but as a seasoned professional healer whose hands and heart have been instrumental in guiding countless individuals towards weight loss triumphs, enriched sexual health, and the surmounting of life's multifaceted challenges to reach the pinnacle of their health aspirations.

My professional and academic journey is a tapestry of diverse yet interconnected disciplines. With an insatiable thirst for knowledge, I delved deep into the realms of yoga and meditation, not just as practices but as academic pursuits, seeking to understand their profound effects on the human psyche and physiology.

This spiritual and intellectual quest further led me to the healing energies of Reiki, the organic wisdom in health foods, and the transformative potential of neuroscience and positive psychology. My foray into the science of health and exercise is not merely academic; it is a reflection of my intrinsic philosophy that the body and mind are inextricable partners in the dance of life.

My dedication to personal growth extends beyond my professional endeavors—it is a way of life. Each morning, as the world stirs awake, I find sanctuary in my daily rituals. My practice of yoga is more than a physical regimen; it is a journey towards achieving a state of zen-like tranquility, a testament to my belief in the power of simplicity and inner peace.Meditation accompanies yoga as my mental compass, guiding me through life's tumultuous waves with a steadfast calm.

What fuels my unyielding passion is an unwavering drive—an innate desire to not only absorb the myriad teachings that life has to offer but also to disseminate them. I am imbued with a relentless drive to unearth and share life strategies that spark a transformative flame within souls, urging them to reach for health, well-being, and the fruition of their deepest dreams.

It was this very desire that led me to the world of writing, to become a scribe of my experiences and insights. My pen is driven by a profound commitment to be a beacon of positivity, influencing the lives of others through words that resonate with truth and vitality.

As you turn the pages of my books, what you will find is a reflection of my heart's work. I invite you into my world, not just as a reader, but as a fellow traveler on this grand adventure of life. Thank you for embarking on this journey with me, and it is my sincerest hope that you will find as much joy in reading my writings as I found in penning them down. May the words you peruse inspire you to cultivate the health and happiness you so richly deserve.

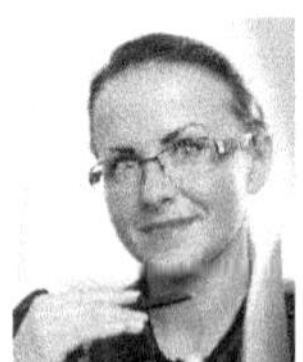

Ashley Fitzgerald

Chapter 1: Understanding Cancer and Its Impacts

Introduction to Cancer: Types, Causes, and Prevalence

Cancer, a word that often brings a chill to the spine, is a complex and multifaceted disease characterized by the uncontrolled growth and spread of abnormal cells in the body. It can develop in virtually any organ or tissue, such as the lung, breast, skin, or bone. The World Health Organization has identified over 100 types of cancers, each with its unique characteristics, behaviors, and treatment responses.

The causes of cancer are varied and often interlinked. They can be broadly classified into genetic factors, lifestyle choices, environmental exposures, and infections. Genetic mutations play a crucial role; some people inherit genes that predispose them to cancer, making them more susceptible to the disease. Lifestyle factors like smoking, excessive alcohol consumption, poor diet, and lack of physical activity significantly increase cancer risk. Environmental exposures to carcinogens, such as asbestos and certain chemicals, and exposure to high levels of radiation are also key contributors. Furthermore, infections from certain viruses, bacteria, or parasites are known to increase the risk of cancer. For instance, human papillomavirus (HPV) is linked to cervical cancer, and hepatitis B and C viruses are linked to liver cancer.

Cancer prevalence varies globally, influenced by factors like age, genetics, lifestyle choices, and environmental exposures. As of the latest global cancer data, the most common cancers include breast, lung, colon, and prostate cancer, affecting millions of people worldwide. The global burden of cancer continues to grow, with significant variations in cancer types and rates across different regions and populations.

Physical and Emotional Impacts of Cancer

The impact of cancer goes beyond the physical realm. Physically, the disease can lead to symptoms like fatigue, pain, weight loss, and changes in body function depending on the cancer type and stage. Treatments like chemotherapy, radiation, and surgery, while often necessary, can have debilitating side effects, including nausea, hair loss, and susceptibility to infections.

Emotionally, the diagnosis of cancer can be overwhelming, leading to a range of feelings from shock and disbelief to fear, anger, and despair. The emotional journey can be as arduous as the physical one, with patients often experiencing anxiety, depression, and a sense of loss of control over their lives. The uncertainty about the future, concerns about body image, and the impact on family and professional life can take a substantial emotional toll.

The emotional impact extends to family members and caregivers, who often undergo significant stress and emotional strain. They may face challenges in providing support, managing their own feelings, and balancing other life responsibilities.

Overview of Traditional and Alternative Cancer Treatments

Traditional cancer treatments are primarily focused on removing or killing cancer cells and typically include surgery, chemotherapy, and radiation therapy. Surgery is often the first line of treatment to remove tumors. Chemotherapy uses drugs to kill rapidly dividing cancer cells but can also affect healthy cells, leading to side effects. Radiation therapy involves using high-energy particles or waves, like X-rays, to destroy or damage cancer cells.

In recent years, targeted therapy and immunotherapy have emerged as significant advances in cancer treatment. Targeted therapy involves drugs that target specific genes or proteins that are involved in cancer cell growth and survival. Immunotherapy helps the body's immune system recognize and attack cancer cells. These therapies are often used in conjunction with traditional treatments and have shown promise in improving outcomes and reducing side effects.

Alongside these medical treatments, there is a growing interest in alternative and complementary therapies. These therapies are used alongside standard treatments to help manage symptoms and improve quality of life. They include practices like acupuncture, massage therapy, herbal remedies, meditation, and yoga. These are not intended to cure cancer but can help manage symptoms and improve overall well-being.

Nutritional therapy is another vital aspect of cancer care. A balanced diet can help maintain strength, reduce treatment side effects, and improve recovery. Nutritionists specializing in cancer care can provide guidance on the best dietary choices during and after treatment.

The field of cancer treatment is continuously evolving, with research and clinical trials constantly seeking new and improved ways to treat and manage the disease. Personalized medicine, where treatment is tailored to the individual characteristics of each patient's cancer, represents the future of cancer care. This approach aims to increase the effectiveness of treatment while minimizing side effects, offering hope for better outcomes and improved quality of life for cancer patients.

In conclusion, understanding cancer's types, causes, and impacts is crucial for patients, families, and healthcare providers. It requires a comprehensive approach that addresses not only the physical aspects of the disease but also the emotional, psychological, and lifestyle factors. As we continue to advance in our understanding and treatment of cancer, a holistic approach that combines traditional and alternative therapies will be essential in providing the best care and support for those affected by this challenging disease.

Chapter 2: Introduction to Somatic Therapy

Definition and History of Somatic Therapy

Somatic Therapy, a term derived from the Greek word 'soma' meaning 'body,' is a holistic therapeutic approach focusing on the integration of mind, body, spirit, and emotions. Its core principle is that the mind and body are interconnected and reciprocal in their impact on one's health and well-being. The roots of somatic therapy can be traced back to the early 20th century, evolving from the work of pioneers like Wilhelm Reich, who emphasized the link between mental health and physical body states, and Elsa Gindler, who developed methods of self-awareness through body movement.

Throughout the decades, various forms of somatic therapy have emerged, including the Alexander Technique, Feldenkrais Method, and Body-Mind Centering. These approaches share the common goal of helping individuals become more aware of their bodily sensations and learn how to release tension and trauma stored in the body. Somatic therapy gained prominence in the latter half of the 20th century, as research began to show the profound impact of trauma and stress on the physical body and overall health.

Principles and Philosophies Behind Somatic Therapy

The foundational principle of somatic therapy is the inseparability of the mind and body. It posits that emotional, psychological, and mental stresses manifest physically in the body, often as chronic pain, tension, or other health issues. Somatic therapists work with clients to identify and release these physical manifestations of emotional distress. The approach is grounded in the belief that through increasing bodily awareness and sensation, individuals can tap into deep-seated emotional experiences and begin the process of healing.

Another key philosophy of somatic therapy is the concept of 'somatic awareness' or 'body mindfulness.' This involves guiding clients to pay attention to bodily sensations and responses, facilitating a deeper understanding of how their bodies hold and express emotions. Techniques like deep breathing, guided imagery, and mindful movement are often used to enhance this awareness.

Central to somatic therapy is the belief in the body's inherent ability to heal itself. The therapist's role is to facilitate this healing process, helping clients to tune into their body's wisdom and learn to trust their body's cues and signals. This empowers individuals to take an active role in their healing journey, fostering a sense of autonomy and self-efficacy.

How Somatic Therapy Differs from Other Therapeutic Approaches

Somatic therapy stands out from traditional psychotherapies in several key ways. While traditional psychotherapy often focuses on cognitive processes and verbal communication, somatic therapy places a significant emphasis on non-verbal experiences and body sensations. It operates under the premise that the body holds onto past traumas and stress, which can manifest physically and influence one's emotional and mental health. Somatic therapy, therefore, incorporates physical techniques and exercises to release this stored tension and trauma

Unlike approaches that solely address the mind or emotions, somatic therapy provides a comprehensive approach to healing that encompasses the whole person. It recognizes that psychological issues cannot be entirely separated from the physical body, and thus, the therapy involves the body as an active participant in the therapeutic process.

Another difference lies in the therapeutic environment. Somatic therapy often involves more movement and physical interaction than traditional talk therapies. Sessions may include movement exercises, hands-on bodywork, or other activities that engage the body directly. This creates a dynamic and interactive therapeutic experience, different from the more static nature of traditional psychotherapy sessions.

Additionally, somatic therapy is deeply rooted in present-moment experiences. It encourages clients to focus on their current bodily sensations and emotional states, rather than solely discussing past events or future concerns. This present-centered approach helps clients develop a deeper awareness and understanding of their current state of being, facilitating immediate and direct engagement with their healing process.

Somatic therapy also differs in its approach to trauma. Traditional therapies often approach trauma primarily through cognitive understanding and verbal processing. In contrast, somatic therapy addresses the physical manifestations of trauma in the body, helping to release it through physical movement and awareness techniques. This can be particularly effective for individuals who have difficulty processing trauma verbally or who experience physical symptoms related to their emotional trauma.

In conclusion, somatic therapy offers a unique and holistic approach to healing, distinct from other therapeutic modalities. By emphasizing the interconnection between mind and body and utilizing physical techniques to address emotional and psychological issues, somatic therapy provides a comprehensive and integrative path to wellness. Its focus on bodily awareness, the inherent healing potential of the body, and the present-moment experience makes it an effective approach for individuals seeking a deeper understanding and resolution of their physical and emotional challenges. As we continue to understand more about the profound connection between our physical bodies and emotional well-being, somatic therapy stands as a pivotal approach in the field of holistic health and healing.

Chapter 3: Somatic Therapy and Cancer Prevention

Role of Somatic Therapy in Cancer Prevention

Somatic therapy, with its focus on the mind-body connection, plays a significant role in cancer prevention. It emphasizes the importance of holistic well-being, acknowledging that mental, emotional, and physical health are deeply interconnected. In the context of cancer prevention, somatic therapy offers tools and techniques to reduce stress, enhance bodily awareness, and promote healthier lifestyle choices, all of which are key factors in reducing the risk of cancer.

Chronic stress has been identified as a significant risk factor for the development of cancer. Prolonged stress can lead to hormonal imbalances and inflammation, weakening the immune system and potentially contributing to the onset and progression of cancer. Somatic therapy addresses this by teaching individuals how to recognize and manage stress effectively. Techniques such as deep breathing, mindfulness, and body scanning are used to bring awareness to stress responses and to develop healthier ways to cope with stress.

Additionally, somatic therapy encourages a heightened sense of body awareness. By becoming more attuned to their bodies, individuals can better understand and respond to their body's needs, whether it's rest, movement, or emotional release. This heightened awareness can lead to earlier detection of physical anomalies, such as lumps or changes in bodily functions, which are key for early cancer detection and prevention.

Techniques and Exercises for Enhancing Body Awareness

One of the core elements of somatic therapy is enhancing body awareness, which is crucial for recognizing and responding to the body's needs and signals. Several techniques and exercises are employed to achieve this heightened awareness:

1. Mindful Breathing:
   This involves focusing on the breath, noticing the rhythm, depth, and quality of each breath. Mindful breathing helps to calm the mind, reduce stress, and bring awareness to the present moment.

2. Body Scanning:
   This technique involves mentally scanning the body from head to toe, noticing any areas of tension, discomfort, or other sensations. Body scanning is a way to become more aware of how emotions and stress manifest physically in the body.

3. Guided Imagery and Visualization:
   These practices involve using the imagination to visualize a peaceful and healing environment or process. This technique can help reduce stress, promote relaxation, and enhance the body's natural healing processes.

4. Movement Therapies:
   Techniques such as yoga, Tai Chi, and dance therapy incorporate gentle movements to improve body awareness, flexibility, and strength. These practices also help in recognizing and releasing stored tension or trauma in the body

5. Mindfulness Practices:
   Activities like meditation and mindful walking encourage individuals to stay present and aware of

their bodily sensations, thoughts, and emotions, fostering a deeper connection between mind and body.

Lifestyle Changes and Habits to Reduce Cancer Risk

In addition to specific techniques, somatic therapy also emphasizes the importance of overall lifestyle changes and habits to reduce cancer risk. These include:

1. Nutritional Awareness:
    Adopting a balanced and nutritious diet is crucial for cancer prevention. This involves consuming a variety of fruits, vegetables, whole grains, and lean proteins, and limiting processed foods, sugars, and unhealthy fats. Somatic therapy encourages mindful eating, where individuals learn to listen to their body's cues for hunger and fullness.

2. Regular Physical Activity:
    Engaging in regular physical activity helps maintain a healthy weight, reduces stress, and improves immune function. Activities can range from brisk walking to more structured exercises like strength training or aerobics.

3. Stress Management:
    Since chronic stress is a risk factor for cancer, managing stress through practices like meditation, deep breathing, and relaxation techniques is an essential part of a cancer-preventive lifestyle.

4. Adequate Rest and Sleep:
    Ensuring sufficient sleep and rest is vital for overall health and cancer prevention. Somatic therapy can help

address sleep disturbances through relaxation techniques and creating a conducive sleep environment.

5. Reducing Exposure to Toxins:
    Minimizing exposure to environmental toxins, such as tobacco smoke, pesticides, and harmful chemicals, is important for reducing cancer risk. Somatic therapy encourages awareness of environmental health and making choices that minimize exposure to these harmful substances.

6. Emotional Well-being:
    Addressing emotional health is key in cancer prevention. Somatic therapy helps individuals process and release negative emotions, develop coping strategies, and foster positive emotional experiences.

7. Social Connections:
    Maintaining strong social connections and support systems is beneficial for mental and emotional health, which in turn can contribute to reduced cancer risk.

In conclusion, somatic therapy offers a comprehensive approach to cancer prevention. By emphasizing the importance of body awareness, stress management, and healthy lifestyle choices, somatic therapy empowers individuals to take proactive steps towards reducing their cancer risk. Through a combination of specific techniques and broader lifestyle changes, somatic therapy provides tools not only for cancer prevention but also for enhancing overall health and well-being As awareness of the mind-body connection continues to grow, somatic therapy stands as a vital approach in the field of

Chapter 4: Somatic Therapy During Cancer Treatment

How Somatic Therapy Can Complement Traditional Cancer Treatments

Somatic therapy, with its holistic approach focusing on the mind-body connection, offers significant benefits as a complementary therapy during cancer treatment. Traditional cancer treatments like chemotherapy, radiation, and surgery, while often necessary for combating the disease, can be physically and emotionally taxing for patients. Somatic therapy steps in to fill gaps that traditional treatments might leave, particularly in managing pain, stress, and the emotional toll of a cancer diagnosis.

One of the key ways somatic therapy complements traditional cancer treatments is through its emphasis on stress reduction. High levels of stress can not only exacerbate the side effects of cancer treatments but also impact the body's ability to heal. Somatic therapy techniques such as deep breathing, mindfulness, and body awareness exercises help in reducing stress and promoting relaxation. This enhanced relaxation can boost the immune system, potentially improving the body's response to cancer treatments.

Another critical aspect is pain management. Many cancer patients experience significant pain, either from the disease itself or as a side effect of treatments. Somatic therapy offers non-pharmacological approaches to pain management, such as guided imagery, mindful movement, and gentle bodywork, which can be effective in reducing perceptions of pain.

Furthermore, somatic therapy aids in addressing the emotional and psychological impacts of cancer. A cancer diagnosis can be a life-altering event, often bringing feelings of fear, anxiety, and depression. Somatic therapy helps patients process these emotions in a healthy way, using body-centered techniques to release emotional tension and improve mental well-being.

Techniques to Manage Pain, Stress, and Side Effects of Cancer Treatments

1. Mindful Breathing:
    This technique involves focusing on slow, deep breaths, which can activate the body's relaxation response and help mitigate stress and anxiety. It can also be particularly effective in managing pain and discomfort during and after treatment sessions.

2. Progressive Muscle Relaxation:
    Progressive muscle relaxation involves tensing and then relaxing different muscle groups in the body. This practice can reduce physical tension and pain and is also beneficial for calming the mind.

3. Guided Imagery and Visualization:
    Patients are guided to envision a calming scene or a healing process within their bodies. This technique can be particularly effective in managing side effects like nausea and fatigue, and in promoting a positive mental state.

4. Movement Therapies:
    Gentle forms of exercise such as yoga, Tai Chi, or Qi Gong can be adapted for cancer patients These practices help in maintaining flexibility, reducing muscle stiffness, and improving circulation, all of which can be affected by cancer treatments.

5. Bodywork and Massage:
   When appropriate, bodywork and massage can be
   integrated into the treatment plan to relieve pain,
   improve lymphatic flow, and provide a sense of comfort
   and care.

Case Studies and Patient Experiences

Case Study 1: Managing Pain and Anxiety during
Chemotherapy

Sarah, a 42-year-old breast cancer patient, experienced high
levels of anxiety and pain during her chemotherapy
treatments. As part of her integrated care plan, she began
somatic therapy, focusing on mindful breathing and guided
imagery. During her chemotherapy sessions, Sarah used these
techniques to manage her anxiety and pain. Over time, she
reported a significant decrease in her anxiety levels and a
better ability to manage pain, making her chemotherapy
experience more manageable.

Case Study 2: Recovering Mobility and Strength Post-Surgery

John, a 60-year-old with colorectal cancer, underwent surgery
that left him with reduced mobility and significant discomfort.
As part of his rehabilitation, he participated in a somatic
therapy program that included gentle movement exercises and
progressive muscle relaxation. Over several weeks, John
regained much of his lost mobility and reported a substantial
decrease in pain levels. The somatic exercises also helped him
develop a more positive outlook towards his recovery.

Patient Experience: Overcoming Emotional Trauma

Linda, diagnosed with ovarian cancer, found the emotional impact of her diagnosis to be overwhelming. Somatic therapy, particularly techniques focusing on emotional release and body awareness, helped her process the trauma associated with her diagnosis. Through somatic therapy, Linda learned how to identify and release emotional tension held in her body, leading to improved emotional well-being and resilience.

In conclusion, somatic therapy offers a valuable complement to traditional cancer treatments. By addressing the physical, emotional, and psychological needs of cancer patients, it provides a more holistic approach to care. The techniques used in somatic therapy can effectively manage pain, reduce stress, and alleviate treatment side effects, enhancing the quality of life for patients undergoing cancer treatment. The case studies and patient experiences highlight the transformative impact somatic therapy can have, not just in managing the symptoms of cancer and its treatments, but in empowering patients to navigate their cancer journey with greater strength and resilience. As the medical community continues to recognize the importance of treating the whole person, somatic therapy stands as a vital component in the comprehensive care of cancer patients.

Chapter 5: Body Awareness and Mindfulness

Deepening Body Awareness through Mindfulness Practices

In the journey of healing and wellness, particularly in the context of cancer treatment, deepening body awareness through mindfulness practices is a crucial aspect. Mindfulness, the practice of being fully present and engaged in the moment, without judgment, helps individuals become more attuned to their bodies. This heightened awareness can lead to better understanding and management of physical and emotional needs, an essential component in the treatment and recovery process for cancer patients.

Mindfulness practices encourage a focused attention on bodily sensations, thoughts, and emotions. This can include observing the breath, noticing areas of tension or relaxation in the body, and acknowledging thoughts and emotions without getting caught up in them. By regularly engaging in these practices, individuals can develop a deeper connection with their bodies, learning to listen and respond to its signals with greater sensitivity and awareness.

For cancer patients, this deepened body awareness is particularly valuable. It can lead to early detection of physical changes or complications, improved management of symptoms and side effects, and a greater sense of control and empowerment over their health and well-being.

Mind-Body Connection and Its Significance in Cancer Treatment

The mind-body connection refers to the powerful interplay between our mental, emotional, and physical states. In the context of cancer treatment, understanding and leveraging this connection is significant. Emotional stress, anxiety, and negative thought patterns can have a tangible impact on physical health, potentially affecting the progression of the disease and the body's response to treatment. Conversely, a positive mindset, emotional resilience, and stress reduction can enhance physical well-being and potentially improve treatment outcomes.

Mindfulness practices play a key role in harnessing the mind-body connection for cancer patients. By fostering a state of relaxation and reducing stress, mindfulness can help mitigate the adverse side effects of cancer treatments such as chemotherapy and radiation. It can also boost the immune system, improve sleep quality, and enhance overall quality of life.

Moreover, mindfulness and body awareness practices can help patients process and cope with the emotional and psychological challenges of a cancer diagnosis. By bringing attention to the present moment and acknowledging thoughts and feelings without judgment, patients can develop healthier coping mechanisms, reduce anxiety and depression, and foster a more positive and hopeful outlook.

Guided Exercises for Mindfulness and Relaxation

1. Mindful Breathing:
   This simple yet powerful exercise involves focusing attention on the breath. Sit or lie in a comfortable position, close your eyes, and bring your attention to your breathing. Notice the sensation of air entering and leaving your nostrils, the rise and fall of your chest or abdomen, and any other sensations that occur as you breathe. Whenever your mind wanders, gently bring

your focus back to your breath. Practice this for 5-10 minutes daily.

2. Body Scan Meditation:
    Begin in a comfortable lying or sitting position. Close your eyes and take a few deep breaths to relax. Start focusing your attention on the top of your head and gradually move down to your toes, paying attention to each part of your body in turn. Notice any sensations, tension, or discomfort in each area. Breathe into these areas and allow them to relax as much as possible. This exercise can be done for 10-20 minutes.

3. Mindful Movement:
    Gentle movement practices like yoga or Tai Chi can be adapted for mindfulness. Focus on the movement of your body and your breath, being present with each pose or form. Notice the sensations in your muscles and joints, and the rhythm of your breath. This practice not only enhances mindfulness but also improves physical strength and flexibility.

4. Guided Imagery:
    Use visualization to promote relaxation and healing. Imagine a peaceful place, such as a beach or a forest. Picture yourself in this place, experiencing it with all your senses – the sights, sounds, smells, and sensations. Guided imagery can be a powerful tool for stress reduction and emotional healing.

5. Mindful Eating:
    This practice involves paying full attention to the experience of eating. Focus on the taste, texture, and smell of your food. Eat slowly, savoring each bite, and listen to your body's hunger and fullness cues. This

practice can improve digestion and promote a healthier relationship with food.

In conclusion, body awareness and mindfulness are invaluable tools in the journey of cancer treatment and recovery. By deepening body awareness and harnessing the mind-body connection, mindfulness practices offer a pathway to greater physical and emotional well-being. These practices not only help manage the side effects of cancer treatment but also empower patients to play an active role in their healing process. As mindfulness and body awareness become integral parts of cancer care, they open doors to a more holistic and patient-centered approach to health and healing.

Chapter 6: Emotional Healing and Trauma Release

Addressing Emotional Trauma Associated with Cancer

The diagnosis and treatment of cancer can be a profoundly traumatic experience, often accompanied by a whirlwind of intense and complex emotions. Patients may grapple with fear, anxiety, anger, sadness, and a sense of loss - loss of health, control, and normalcy in life. This emotional trauma, if unaddressed, can deeply impact the quality of life and even the efficacy of medical treatments.

Cancer-related emotional trauma can manifest in various ways. Some individuals may experience persistent anxiety and fear, especially concerning the uncertainty of their disease's outcome. Others may face depression, feeling overwhelmed by the changes and challenges brought on by their illness. Moreover, the trauma can extend to the patient's family and caregivers, who also face emotional burdens.

Recognizing and addressing this emotional trauma is a critical component of comprehensive cancer care. It involves acknowledging the emotional impact of the disease, providing support and resources to cope with these challenges, and implementing strategies to process and release these deep-seated emotions.

Techniques for Emotional Release and Healing

1. Somatic Experiencing:
   This approach involves focusing on bodily sensations and movements to release and resolve the physical manifestations of trauma. Through guided exercises, patients learn to identify tension and discomfort in their

bodies related to emotional stress and to use specific techniques to release this tension.

2. Expressive Arts Therapy:
    Activities like painting, drawing, writing, or music allow patients to express emotions that might be difficult to articulate verbally. These creative outlets offer a way to explore and process feelings in a therapeutic and non-threatening manner.

3. Mindfulness and Meditation:
    Practices like mindfulness meditation help patients stay present and aware of their emotions without becoming overwhelmed by them. Through regular practice, patients can develop a more balanced perspective, reducing anxiety and depression.

4. Guided Imagery and Visualization:
    This technique involves using the imagination to visualize a peaceful and healing environment or process. It can help reduce stress, promote relaxation, and support emotional healing.

5. Breathwork:
    Controlled breathing exercises can be a powerful tool for managing emotional distress. Techniques like diaphragmatic breathing help regulate the stress response and promote a sense of calm and relaxation.

6. Journaling:
    Writing about thoughts, feelings, and experiences can be therapeutic. It provides an outlet for expressing emotions and can help patients process their feelings and gain insights into their emotional state.

7. Support Groups and Peer Support:
    Sharing experiences with others who have gone
    through similar situations can be incredibly validating
    and comforting. Support groups provide a safe space to
    express emotions, share coping strategies, and foster a
    sense of community and understanding.

Importance of Psychological Support During Cancer Treatment

The role of psychological support in cancer treatment cannot be overstated. It is essential for managing the emotional and mental health challenges that accompany a cancer diagnosis. Psychological support can take many forms, including individual counseling, support groups, family therapy, and psychoeducational interventions.

Individual counseling provides a private and safe space for patients to discuss their fears, concerns, and emotions with a trained professional. This can help them develop coping strategies, address any underlying mental health issues like anxiety or depression, and navigate the complex emotional landscape of their cancer journey.

Support groups offer a sense of community and belonging, helping patients feel less isolated in their experiences. These groups can provide practical advice, emotional support, and the opportunity to share experiences and coping strategies with others who understand what they are going through.

Family therapy can be crucial, as cancer affects not just the patient but their entire family. This form of therapy helps families communicate effectively, support each other, and manage the stress and emotional burden that cancer can bring.

Psychoeducational interventions provide patients and their families with information about cancer, its treatment, and strategies to manage the psychological impact of the disease. This knowledge can empower patients and their families, reducing anxiety and helping them feel more in control.

In conclusion, emotional healing and trauma release are vital aspects of cancer care. Addressing the emotional trauma associated with cancer and providing comprehensive psychological support can significantly improve patients' quality of life and even impact their treatment outcomes. Techniques such as somatic experiencing, expressive arts therapy, mindfulness, and breathwork, along with psychological support through counseling and support groups, offer effective ways to manage and process the complex emotions associated with cancer. By integrating these approaches into cancer care, we can offer patients a more holistic and compassionate path to healing and recovery.

Chapter 7: Physical Exercises and Movement Therapy

Role of Physical Activity in Cancer Recovery and Prevention

Physical activity plays a critical role in both the prevention and recovery process for cancer patients. Research has consistently shown that regular exercise can reduce the risk of developing certain types of cancer, including breast, colon, and endometrial cancers. For those undergoing or recovering from cancer treatment, physical activity offers numerous benefits, such as improving physical function, reducing fatigue, and enhancing overall quality of life. Additionally, regular exercise can boost mental health, reduce the risk of cancer recurrence, and improve survival rates for certain types of cancer.

Engaging in physical activity during and after cancer treatment can help mitigate some of the side effects of treatments such as chemotherapy, radiation therapy, and surgery. Exercise can help combat fatigue, improve muscle strength and endurance, maintain a healthy weight, and enhance mood and self-esteem. It can also improve cardiovascular health, which may be compromised due to certain cancer treatments.

Specific Somatic Exercises and Movement Therapies

1. Gentle Aerobic Exercise:
   Activities like walking, cycling, or swimming are excellent for improving cardiovascular health and enhancing mood. These low-impact exercises can be adapted to various fitness levels and can be gradually increased in intensity and duration as the patient's strength and endurance improve.

2. Strength Training:
   Resistance exercises, using weights or resistance bands, can help rebuild muscle strength and bone density, which may be affected by cancer treatments. Strength training should be tailored to the individual's abilities and should focus on major muscle groups.

3. Yoga and Tai Chi:
   These practices combine gentle movements, stretching, and breath control. They are particularly beneficial for improving flexibility, balance, and relaxation. Yoga and Tai Chi can also help in managing stress, anxiety, and fatigue.

4. Pilates:
   Pilates focuses on strengthening the core muscles, improving posture, and increasing flexibility. It is particularly effective in rebuilding strength and stability, especially for patients who have undergone surgeries that affect the abdomen, breast, or other core areas.

5. Dance Therapy:
   Dance therapy uses choreographed or free-form movement to express emotions and improve physical strength and coordination. It can be an enjoyable way to exercise and has been shown to improve emotional well-being.

6. Aquatic Therapy:
   Exercising in water provides a low-impact environment that is gentle on the joints. Aquatic therapy can be especially beneficial for those with lymphedema, a common side effect of some cancer treatments.

Tailoring Exercises to Individual Needs and Limitations

When incorporating physical exercises and movement therapy into a cancer recovery and prevention plan, it is crucial to tailor these activities to each individual's needs, limitations, and current health status. Here are some considerations:

1. Consult Healthcare Providers:
   Before starting any exercise regimen, it's important for cancer patients to consult with their healthcare team. This includes discussing the type of cancer, the treatments received, and any side effects or complications. This information will help in designing a safe and effective exercise program.

2. Start Slowly:
   For many cancer patients, especially those currently undergoing treatment or in the early stages of recovery, energy levels and physical abilities may be limited. Starting with short, low-intensity sessions and gradually increasing the duration and intensity is key.

3. Consider Existing Limitations:
   Each individual's limitations should be taken into account. For example, patients with neuropathy may need to avoid high-impact activities, while those with lymphedema may benefit from specialized exercises to reduce swelling.

4. Monitor Response to Exercise:
   It's important to closely monitor how the body responds to exercise. This includes paying attention to any new or worsening symptoms and adjusting the exercise program accordingly.

5. Incorporate Variety:
    Including a variety of exercises can help address different aspects of physical fitness, such as strength, flexibility, and endurance, and can also keep the exercise program engaging and enjoyable.

6. Seek Professional Guidance:
    Working with professionals like physiotherapists, exercise physiologists, or certified cancer exercise trainers can be extremely beneficial. These experts can help design a personalized exercise program, teach proper techniques, and provide motivation and support.

In conclusion, physical exercises and movement therapy are integral components of cancer recovery and prevention. They offer numerous benefits, ranging from physical to emotional well-being. By carefully tailoring exercise programs to individual needs and limitations, and with appropriate guidance and support, cancer patients can safely engage in physical activities that enhance their recovery process and overall quality of life. As the field of cancer care continues to evolve, the integration of physical exercises and movement therapy into treatment plans signifies a shift towards more holistic, patient-centered care.

Chapter 8: Nutrition and Lifestyle in Somatic Therapy

Impact of Diet and Nutrition on Cancer and Recovery

Diet and nutrition play a pivotal role in both cancer prevention and recovery. A healthy diet can reduce the risk of developing certain types of cancer and support the body during and after cancer treatment. Nutritious foods provide the essential vitamins, minerals, and other nutrients that the body needs to maintain strength, repair tissue, and support the immune system.

For cancer patients, proper nutrition is crucial as it helps to manage side effects of treatment, maintain a healthy weight, preserve lean body mass, and improve energy levels. Certain treatments can lead to loss of appetite, changes in taste or smell, nausea, and other digestive issues, making it challenging to maintain adequate nutrition. Tailoring the diet to address these challenges is a key component of cancer care.

Somatic Approach to Eating and Food Choices

The somatic approach to eating goes beyond simply choosing healthy foods; it involves developing a deeper connection with the body and its cues related to hunger, satiety, and nutritional needs. This approach encourages mindfulness in eating – paying attention to the experience of eating, savoring food, and being attuned to the body's signals.

1. Mindful Eating:
   This practice involves eating slowly and without distraction, tuning into the sensory experience of eating, and listening to the body's cues for hunger and fullness. Mindful eating helps in making more conscious food

choices and can improve digestion and satisfaction with meals.

2. Intuitive Eating:
    This is about trusting the body's innate wisdom to guide food choices and eating habits. It means eating in response to physiological hunger cues rather than emotional or external cues and requires a shift from rigid dietary rules to a more flexible, gentle approach to nutrition.

3. Nutrient-Dense Foods:
    Emphasizing whole, minimally processed foods rich in vitamins, minerals, and antioxidants is a cornerstone of the somatic approach. These include fruits, vegetables, whole grains, lean proteins, and healthy fats, which support the body's healing processes.

4. Anti-inflammatory Foods:
    Chronic inflammation can contribute to the development and progression of cancer. Including anti-inflammatory foods such as leafy greens, fatty fish, nuts, and seeds can help reduce inflammation in the body.

5. Hydration:
    Proper hydration is essential for overall health and can be particularly important during cancer treatment to help manage side effects and support bodily functions.

Integrating Healthy Lifestyle Choices for Holistic Healing

A holistic approach to healing from cancer involves integrating various healthy lifestyle choices. These choices support not only physical health but also emotional and mental well-being.

1. Regular Physical Activity:
    As discussed in previous chapters, regular exercise is crucial. It enhances physical strength, boosts mood, and improves energy levels. The type and intensity of exercise should be tailored to each individual's abilities and health status.

2. Stress Management Techniques:
    Stress can negatively impact health and hinder recovery. Techniques such as meditation, yoga, deep breathing exercises, and relaxation techniques are important for managing stress.

3. Adequate Sleep and Rest:
    Quality sleep is essential for healing and recovery. Good sleep hygiene, including maintaining a regular sleep schedule and creating a restful environment, can improve sleep quality.

4. Limiting Alcohol and Avoiding Tobacco:
    Alcohol consumption and tobacco use are known risk factors for many types of cancer. Limiting alcohol intake and avoiding tobacco in all forms is crucial for cancer prevention and recovery.

5. Social Connections and Support:
    Maintaining strong social connections and seeking support from friends, family, or support groups can improve mental and emotional well-being during the cancer journey.

6. Environmental Considerations:
    Reducing exposure to environmental toxins, such as chemicals in cleaning and personal care products, and

prioritizing organic foods when possible, can help reduce the body's toxic burden.

7. Emotional Health:
   Addressing emotional health through therapy, counseling, or other supportive measures is an important aspect of holistic healing.

8. Spiritual Practices:
   For many, spiritual or religious practices can provide comfort, hope, and a sense of peace during cancer treatment and recovery.

In conclusion, integrating nutrition and lifestyle choices is a vital component of somatic therapy in the context of cancer and recovery. A balanced, nutrient-rich diet, combined with healthy lifestyle choices, forms the foundation for holistic healing. This approach not only addresses the physical aspects of recovery but also supports emotional and mental health, offering a comprehensive pathway to wellness. By empowering individuals to make informed choices about their diet and lifestyle, somatic therapy contributes to a more proactive and self-directed journey through cancer treatment and recovery.

Chapter 9: Building a Supportive Community

The Importance of Community and Social Support

In the journey of cancer treatment and recovery, the role of community and social support cannot be overstated. Facing cancer can be an isolating experience, filled with challenges that are difficult to navigate alone. The support of a community – whether it's made up of family, friends, healthcare providers, or fellow patients – provides emotional sustenance, practical assistance, and a sense of belonging that are crucial during this time.

The benefits of social support in cancer care are well-documented. A strong support system can improve psychological well-being, reduce symptoms of depression and anxiety, and even positively impact physical health outcomes. Patients who feel supported are often more engaged in their treatment, more motivated to follow through with medical recommendations, and more proactive in their self-care.

Creating and Participating in Support Groups

Support groups are a vital component of the cancer support community. They provide a safe and understanding space where individuals can share experiences, offer advice, and provide emotional support to each other. These groups can be disease-specific, treatment-specific, or open to all cancer patients and survivors.

1. Forming Support Groups:
    Creating a support group can start with a few individuals who share similar experiences. Hospitals, community centers, and religious institutions often provide space for such groups. Online platforms can

also be used to facilitate virtual meetings, broadening the reach to those unable to attend in person.

2. Facilitating Group Meetings:
    Effective support groups often have a facilitator – either a healthcare professional, a trained counselor, or a cancer survivor – who guides the discussion, ensures that everyone has a chance to speak, and maintains a supportive and respectful environment.

3. Incorporating Educational Components:
    Apart from sharing personal experiences, support groups can also provide educational resources, inviting healthcare professionals to speak on relevant topics, or sharing the latest research and information about cancer treatment and recovery.

4. Online Communities:
    For those unable to attend in-person meetings, online forums and social media groups offer an alternative platform for connection and support.

Family, Friends, and Caregiver Roles in Somatic Therapy

The role of family, friends, and caregivers is integral in the somatic therapy process. They are often the primary source of emotional support and practical help, and their involvement can significantly impact the patient's healing journey.

1. Understanding the Patient's Needs:
    Education about somatic therapy and its benefits can help family members and caregivers understand the patient's needs and the importance of body-mind integration in the healing process.

2. Providing Emotional Support:
   A key role of family and friends is to provide emotional support – listening, offering words of encouragement, and being present. This support is invaluable in helping patients cope with the emotional toll of cancer.

3. Participating in Therapy Sessions:
   Sometimes, family members or caregivers may be invited to participate in therapy sessions. This can help them understand the patient's experiences and learn techniques to support them at home.

4. Encouraging Healthy Lifestyle Choices:
   Caregivers and family members can play a significant role in encouraging and facilitating healthy lifestyle choices, such as preparing nutritious meals or participating in physical activities together.

5. Respecting Boundaries:
   It's important for caregivers and family members to respect the patient's boundaries and need for independence. Balancing assistance with respect for the patient's autonomy is crucial.

6. Seeking Support for Themselves:
   Caregiving can be emotionally and physically draining. It's important for caregivers and family members to also seek support for themselves, whether through their own support groups, counseling, or other resources.

7. Maintaining Open Communication:
   Open and honest communication helps in understanding the patient's needs, fears, and expectations, and in providing the appropriate level of support and care.

8. Promoting Positivity and Hope:
    Maintaining a positive environment and fostering hope
    can significantly impact the patient's outlook and
    motivation throughout their cancer journey.

In conclusion, building a supportive community is a
fundamental aspect of cancer care and somatic therapy. The
benefits of social support – whether from support groups,
family, friends, or caregivers – are multifaceted, extending
beyond emotional support to tangible improvements in
treatment adherence and overall health outcomes. By fostering
connections, sharing experiences, and providing support, this
community becomes an invaluable resource in the patient's
journey toward healing and recovery. The integration of social
support into cancer care highlights the importance of treating
the patient not just as an individual, but as a part of a broader
community, each member contributing to the holistic well-
being and recovery of the patient.

Chapter 10: Continuing the Journey

Long-Term Strategies for Maintaining Health and Preventing Recurrence

As patients transition from active cancer treatment to post-treatment life, the focus shifts to maintaining health and preventing recurrence. This phase involves integrating long-term strategies into everyday life, ensuring that the journey towards healing and wellness continues.

1. Adopting a Healthy Lifestyle:
   Continuing the practices of a healthy diet, regular physical activity, and adequate rest is essential. These habits not only contribute to overall well-being but also play a crucial role in reducing the risk of cancer recurrence.

2. Regular Monitoring and Health Check-Ups:
   Regular follow-up appointments with healthcare providers are vital for monitoring health and detecting any signs of recurrence early. Patients should be vigilant about any new symptoms and report them promptly.

3. Continued Stress Management:
   Chronic stress can impact immune function and overall health. Techniques such as mindfulness meditation, yoga, and deep breathing should remain a regular part of life to manage stress effectively.

4. Community Engagement:
   Staying connected with support groups or community networks can provide ongoing emotional support and motivation. These connections also keep individuals

informed about new developments in cancer care and somatic therapy.

5. Lifelong Learning and Adaptation:
    As research in cancer care and somatic therapy evolves, staying informed about new findings and integrating relevant practices into daily life can be beneficial.

Personal Stories of Transformation and Healing

Personal stories of transformation and healing play a powerful role in inspiring and guiding others on a similar journey. These narratives often highlight the resilience of the human spirit and the capacity for growth and healing, even in the face of adversity.

1. Survivor Stories:
    Stories from cancer survivors who have integrated somatic therapy into their recovery can offer hope and practical insights. These narratives can serve as powerful testaments to the effectiveness of holistic approaches in cancer care.

2. Caregiver Perspectives:
    Accounts from caregivers can provide a different but equally important perspective, offering insights into the challenges and rewards of supporting a loved one through cancer treatment and recovery.

3. Professional Insights:
    Healthcare professionals and therapists can share stories of patients who have benefited from somatic therapy, providing a clinical perspective on the transformative power of these approaches.

Resources and Guidance for Further Exploration in Somatic Therapy

For those wishing to explore somatic therapy further, whether as patients, caregivers, or healthcare professionals, a wealth of resources is available.

1. Books and Publications:
   Numerous books and academic publications provide in-depth information on somatic therapy, its techniques, and its applications in cancer care.

2. Online Resources:
   Websites, online forums, and social media groups can be valuable sources of information and support. They offer a platform for sharing experiences, asking questions, and staying updated on the latest research.

3. Workshops and Seminars:
   Participating in workshops or seminars led by experts in somatic therapy can provide hands-on experience and deeper understanding.

4. Professional Training Programs:
   For those interested in practicing somatic therapy, professional training programs offer the necessary education and certification.

5. Local Support Groups and Community Centers:
   These can be resources for finding local therapists, joining support groups, or participating in community events related to somatic therapy and cancer care.

6. Healthcare Providers:

Oncologists, therapists, and counselors can often provide referrals or recommendations for somatic therapy practitioners and resources.

In conclusion, "Continuing the Journey" emphasizes the importance of long-term strategies for maintaining health and preventing cancer recurrence. It underscores the role of personal stories in inspiring and guiding others and highlights the wealth of resources available for further exploration in somatic therapy. This chapter serves as a reminder that the journey of healing and wellness is ongoing, and with the right tools, support, and information, individuals can continue to thrive and maintain their health long after the completion of cancer treatment. The journey through and beyond cancer can be transformative, leading not only to physical healing but also to profound personal growth and a deeper understanding of health and wellness.

Chapter 11. Case studies

Case Study 1: Breast Cancer

Patient: Maria, 45 years old
Cancer Type: Stage II Breast Cancer
Somatic Therapy Used: Yoga and Mindful Breathing
Outcome: Maria underwent a lumpectomy followed by radiation therapy. During her treatment, she started practicing yoga and mindful breathing exercises to manage stress and fatigue. These practices helped her maintain her flexibility, reduced lymphedema symptoms, and enhanced her overall well-being. Post-treatment, Maria reported feeling more in control of her body and emotions, and her follow-up assessments showed good physical recovery and emotional resilience.

Case Study 2: Prostate Cancer

Patient: John, 68 years old
Cancer Type: Stage I Prostate Cancer
Somatic Therapy Used: Tai Chi and Guided Imagery
Outcome: After his diagnosis, John opted for active surveillance with regular check-ups. To manage his anxiety and maintain physical health, he began practicing Tai Chi and guided imagery. These practices improved his balance, strength, and mental focus. John reported a significant reduction in stress levels and an improved sense of wellbeing. His prostate-specific antigen (PSA) levels remained stable, indicating effective management of his condition.

Case Study 3: Lung Cancer

Patient: Angela, 58 years old
Cancer Type: Stage IIIA Non-Small Cell Lung Cancer

Somatic Therapy Used: Breathwork and Body Scanning
Meditation
Outcome: Angela received chemotherapy and targeted therapy.
She experienced significant anxiety and breathlessness.
Integrating breathwork and body scanning meditation into her
routine helped Angela manage her symptoms. These practices
improved her lung capacity, reduced anxiety, and helped her
cope with the side effects of treatment. Over time, Angela's
follow-up scans showed a reduction in tumor size, and her
quality of life significantly improved.

Case Study 4: Colorectal Cancer

Patient: David, 50 years old
Cancer Type: Stage IIB Colorectal Cancer
Somatic Therapy Used: Pilates and Progressive Muscle
Relaxation
Outcome: Post-surgery and during chemotherapy, David
suffered from fatigue and muscle weakness. He started Pilates
and progressive muscle relaxation exercises to strengthen his
core muscles and manage pain. These exercises improved his
posture, digestion, and energy levels. David reported feeling
stronger and more energetic, and his recovery process was
smoother than expected. His post-treatment evaluations
showed no signs of recurrence.

Case Study 5: Ovarian Cancer

Patient: Sarah, 38 years old
Cancer Type: Stage IIIC Ovarian Cancer
Somatic Therapy Used: Dance Therapy and Mindfulness
Outcome: Sarah underwent surgery and chemotherapy. She
experienced emotional distress and physical discomfort.
Joining a dance therapy group and practicing mindfulness
helped her express her emotions and regain physical strength.

Sarah found a supportive community in the dance group, which improved her mood and self-esteem. Her post-treatment scans showed no evidence of disease, and she continued dance therapy as part of her long-term wellness plan.

These case studies illustrate the effectiveness of somatic therapy in complementing traditional cancer treatments. By addressing the physical and emotional needs of patients, somatic therapy can enhance the quality of life, aid in recovery, and contribute to the overall management of cancer.

Chapter 12. Weekly activities schedule
-Exercises plan
-Food plan

Weekly exercises schedule

Creating a weekly life schedule incorporating various techniques recommended for somatic therapy in cancer healing and control can be a valuable tool for patients. This schedule aims to balance different practices like mindfulness, physical exercises, nutrition, and relaxation techniques, ensuring a comprehensive approach to well-being. The schedule below is a general template and should be adapted to individual needs, preferences, and medical advice.

This schedule is designed to provide a balanced approach to incorporating somatic therapy techniques into daily life, promoting healing and well-being for individuals recovering from or managing cancer.

Monday
- 7:00 AM: Mindful Breathing (10 min)
- 7:30 AM: Healthy Breakfast
- 8:30 AM: Gentle Walk (30 min)
- 10:00 AM: Somatic Exercise Session (45 min)
- 12:00 PM: Mindful Eating Lunch
- 2:00 PM: Body Scan Meditation (20 min)
- 4:00 PM: Nutrition Workshop / Cooking Class
- 6:00 PM: Healthy Dinner
- 8:00 PM: Progressive Muscle Relaxation (20 min)
- 9:00 PM: Journaling / Reflective Time (15 min)
- 10:00 PM: Prepare for Bed / Quiet Time

Tuesday
- 7:00 AM: Mindful Breathing (10 min)

- 7:30 AM: Healthy Breakfast
- 8:30 AM: Tai Chi (30 min)
- 10:00 AM: Guided Imagery (20 min)
- 12:00 PM: Mindful Eating Lunch
- 2:00 PM: Pilates (30 min)
- 4:00 PM: Support Group Meeting
- 6:00 PM: Healthy Dinner
- 8:00 PM: Dance Therapy Session (45 min)
- 9:00 PM: Journaling / Reflective Time (15 min)
- 10:00 PM: Prepare for Bed / Quiet Time

Wednesday
- 7:00 AM: Mindful Breathing (10 min)
- 7:30 AM: Healthy Breakfast
- 8:30 AM: Gentle Walk (30 min)
- 10:00 AM: Somatic Exercise Session (45 min)
- 12:00 PM: Mindful Eating Lunch
- 2:00 PM: Body Scan Meditation (20 min)
- 4:00 PM: Nutrition Workshop / Cooking Class
- 6:00 PM: Healthy Dinner
- 8:00 PM: Progressive Muscle Relaxation (20 min)
- 9:00 PM: Journaling / Reflective Time (15 min)
- 10:00 PM: Prepare for Bed / Quiet Time

Thursday
- 7:00 AM: Mindful Breathing (10 min)
- 7:30 AM: Healthy Breakfast
- 8:30 AM: Yoga (30 min)
- 10:00 AM: Guided Imagery (20 min)
- 12:00 PM: Mindful Eating Lunch
- 2:00 PM: Pilates (30 min)
- 4:00 PM: Support Group Meeting
- 6:00 PM: Healthy Dinner
- 8:00 PM: Dance Therapy Session (45 min)
- 9:00 PM: Journaling / Reflective Time (15 min)

- 10:00 PM: Prepare for Bed / Quiet Time

Friday
- 7:00 AM: Mindful Breathing (10 min)
- 7:30 AM: Healthy Breakfast
- 8:30 AM: Gentle Walk (30 min)
- 10:00 AM: Somatic Exercise Session (45 min)
- 12:00 PM: Mindful Eating Lunch
- 2:00 PM: Body Scan Meditation (20 min)
- 4:00 PM: Nutrition Workshop / Cooking Class
- 6:00 PM: Healthy Dinner
- 8:00 PM: Progressive Muscle Relaxation (20 min)
- 9:00 PM: Journaling / Reflective Time (15 min)
- 10:00 PM: Prepare for Bed / Quiet Time

Saturday
- 7:00 AM: Sleep In / Rest
- 7:30 AM: Healthy Breakfast
- 8:30 AM: Yoga (45 min)
- 10:00 AM: Creative Activity (e.g., Art Therapy)
- 12:00 PM: Mindful Eating Lunch
- 2:00 PM: Free Time / Rest
- 4:00 PM: Outdoor Activity (e.g., Gardening)
- 6:00 PM: Healthy Dinner
- 8:00 PM: Movie Night / Social Gathering
- 9:00 PM: Journaling / Reflective Time (15 min)
- 10:00 PM: Prepare for Bed / Quiet Time

Sunday
- 7:00 AM: Sleep In / Rest
- 7:30 AM: Healthy Breakfast
- 8:30 AM: Family Time / Leisure Activities
- 10:00 AM: Brunch / Leisure Activity
- 12:00 PM: Mindful Eating Lunch
- 2:00 PM: Free Time / Rest

- 4:00 PM: Outdoor Activity (e.g., Nature Walk)
- 6:00 PM: Healthy Dinner

Flexibility:
This schedule is a guideline and should be adjusted based on personal energy levels, medical appointments, and individual preferences.

Rest:
Adequate rest is crucial. If any activity feels too strenuous, it should be skipped or replaced with a restful activity.

Nutrition:
Emphasis on balanced, nutritious meals. Consulting with a nutritionist for personalized meal planning can be beneficial.

Social and Emotional Well-being:
Incorporating social activities and time for emotional reflection is important for holistic healing.

Professional Guidance:
For specific exercises and therapies, working with professionals is recommended to ensure they are done safely and effectively.

Hydration: Regular hydration throughout the day is important, especially on days with more physical activities.
-

Creating a week-long healthy meal plan to accompany the somatic therapy schedule can enhance overall wellness and support the healing process. The following meal plan is designed to provide balanced nutrition with a focus on cancer recovery and prevention. This is a general guide and should be adjusted to individual dietary needs and preferences.

Weekly Food plan

Monday
- Breakfast: Oatmeal with fresh berries, almonds, and a drizzle of honey.
- Lunch: Grilled chicken salad with mixed greens, cherry tomatoes, cucumber, and avocado. Olive oil and lemon dressing.
- Dinner: Baked salmon with steamed broccoli and quinoa.

Tuesday
- Breakfast: Greek yogurt with granola and sliced banana.
- Lunch: Whole-grain wrap with turkey, spinach, bell peppers, and hummus.
- Dinner: Stir-fried tofu with mixed vegetables (carrots, snap peas, bell peppers) and brown rice.

Wednesday
- Breakfast: Smoothie with spinach, banana, blueberries, flaxseeds, and almond milk.
- Lunch: Lentil soup with a side of whole-grain bread.
- Dinner: Grilled lean steak, sweet potato, and a side salad with mixed greens.

Thursday
- Breakfast: Scrambled eggs with spinach, mushrooms, and whole-grain toast.
- Lunch: Quinoa salad with black beans, corn, cherry tomatoes, and cilantro. Lime vinaigrette.
- Dinner: Baked chicken breast with roasted Brussels sprouts and wild rice.

Friday
- Breakfast: Whole-grain cereal with skim milk and a side of mixed fruit.

- Lunch: Tuna salad with mixed greens, red onion, and whole-grain crackers.
- Dinner: Vegetable stir-fry with shrimp and brown rice.

Saturday
- Breakfast: Whole-grain pancakes topped with fresh berries and a small amount of maple syrup.
- Lunch: Caprese salad (fresh mozzarella, tomatoes, basil) with balsamic reduction and a side of whole-grain bread.
- Dinner: Grilled vegetable kebabs (bell peppers, zucchini, mushrooms, cherry tomatoes) with grilled chicken and couscous.

Sunday
- Breakfast: Avocado toast on whole-grain bread with a poached egg and a side of fruit.
- Lunch: Grilled salmon salad with mixed greens, cucumber, and avocado. Lemon and olive oil dressing.
- Dinner: Roasted chicken with mixed roasted vegetables (carrots, parsnips, beets).

Snacks (can be enjoyed as needed throughout the day):
- Fresh fruit (apples, berries, oranges, grapes).
- Raw nuts (almonds, walnuts, pecans).
- Carrot and celery sticks with hummus.
- Greek yogurt with a sprinkle of chia seeds.
- Whole-grain crackers with cheese or nut butter.

Hydration:
- Aim to drink at least 8 glasses of water per day.
- Herbal teas and infused water with lemon or cucumber for variety.

This meal plan focuses on incorporating a variety of fruits, vegetables, whole grains, lean proteins, and healthy fats, all of which are key components of a diet that supports cancer recovery and overall health. Before making any significant changes to your diet, especially if you have specific health conditions or dietary needs, it's important to consult with a healthcare provider or a registered dietitian.

Chapter 13. References
-Book list
-Academic Open Access Journals
-Searching key words

Book list

These books typically explore how mind-body practices and techniques can aid in the healing process for cancer patients, offering insights into managing physical and emotional well-being. Here's a list of books that might be relevant to this topic:

1. "The Body Keeps the Score: Brain, Mind, and Body in the Healing of Trauma" by Bessel van der Kolk - While not exclusively about cancer, this book provides a comprehensive look at how trauma affects the body and mind, and how somatic therapy can aid in healing.

2. "Waking the Tiger: Healing Trauma" by Peter A. Levine - Levine's work in somatic experiencing offers valuable insights into understanding and healing trauma, which can be relevant for cancer patients dealing with the emotional and psychological impact of their illness.

3. "Molecules of Emotion: The Science Behind Mind-Body Medicine" by Candace B. Pert - This book delves into the connection between the mind and body and how emotions can impact physical health, offering perspectives that could be applied to cancer healing.

4. "Healing Trauma: A Pioneering Program for Restoring the Wisdom of Your Body" by Peter A. Levine - Another work by Levine, this book provides practical guidance and exercises based on somatic experiencing, which can be beneficial for those undergoing cancer treatment.

5. "Mind Over Medicine: Scientific Proof That You Can Heal Yourself" by Lissa Rankin, MD - This book explores the science behind how thoughts and emotions can affect physical health, including in the context of serious illnesses like cancer.

6. "Radical Remission: Surviving Cancer Against All Odds" by Kelly A. Turner, Ph.D. - Turner's research on cancer patients who have experienced remissions offers insights into various factors that can contribute to healing, including mind-body practices.

7. "Anti-Cancer: A New Way of Life" by David Servan-Schreiber - Servan-Schreiber, a doctor and brain cancer survivor, combines personal experience and scientific research to explore how lifestyle changes, including mental and emotional aspects, can contribute to cancer healing.

8. "Love, Medicine and Miracles" by Bernie S. Siegel, MD - Dr. Siegel's work focuses on the powerful effects of the mind on the body, especially in the context of fighting cancer.

9. "Full Catastrophe Living: Using the Wisdom of Your Body and Mind to Face Stress, Pain, and Illness" by Jon Kabat-Zinn - This book, while broader in its scope, includes techniques like mindfulness-based stress reduction that can be highly beneficial for cancer patients.

10. "When the Body Says No: Exploring the Stress-Disease Connection" by Gabor Maté - Dr. Maté explores how chronic stress and emotional repression can impact physical health, including the development and progression of diseases like cancer.

These books offer a range of perspectives on the connection between mind, body, and health, and provide valuable resources for those interested in exploring somatic therapy as a complementary approach to cancer treatment and recovery.

Academic Open Access Journals

Notable open access journals that are known for publishing high-quality, peer-reviewed academic research in various fields. While these journals cover a broad range of topics, many of them include studies related to health, nutrition, medicine, and related sciences, which would encompass research on topics like food and hypertension:

1. PLOS ONE (Public Library of Science ONE)
   - Covers a wide range of scientific disciplines including life sciences, environmental sciences, and health sciences.
(https://www.plosone.org/)

2. BMJ Open
   - An online, open access journal, dedicated to publishing medical research from all disciplines and therapeutic areas.
 (https://bmjopen.bmj.com/)

3. Frontiers
   - A leading open access publisher with journals covering a wide array of academic disciplines, including health, nutrition, and medicine.
(https://www.frontiersin.org/)

4. BioMed Central (BMC)
   - Offers a large portfolio of peer-reviewed open access journals, encompassing all areas of biology, biomedicine, and medicine.
(https://www.biomedcentral.com/)

5. MDPI (Multidisciplinary Digital Publishing Institute)
  - Publishes a wide range of open access journals including "Nutrients", which focuses on human nutrition.
(https://www.mdpi.com/)

6. Hindawi
  - Publishes peer-reviewed, open access journals covering a wide range of academic disciplines including medicine and health sciences.
 (https://www.hindawi.com/)

7. eLife
  - An open access journal that publishes research in the life sciences and biomedicine.
 (https://elifesciences.org/)

8. Scientific Reports (Nature Publishing Group)
  - An open access journal publishing original research from all areas of the natural and clinical sciences.
 (https://www.nature.com/srep/)

9. JAMA Network Open
  - An international open access journal publishing clinical care, health policy, and global health research.
(https://jamanetwork.com/journals/jamanetworkopen)

10. The Lancet Digital Health
  - A gold open access journal in the Lancet family, dedicated to digital health and health informatics.
(https://www.thelancet.com/digital-health)

Searching key words

Here are some types of academic papers you might look for in scholarly databases:

1. Clinical Trials Evaluating Somatic Therapies in Cancer Care: These studies typically involve the implementation of specific somatic therapies (like mindfulness, yoga, tai chi, etc.) in a cohort of cancer patients, assessing outcomes such as pain management, stress reduction, and quality of life.

2. Systematic Reviews and Meta-Analyses: Papers that compile and analyze data from multiple studies on somatic therapies in cancer care, offering a broader perspective on their effectiveness and potential applications.

3. Case Studies: Detailed reports of individual cancer patients' experiences with somatic therapy, highlighting specific therapeutic approaches and outcomes.

4. Qualitative Studies on Patient Experiences: Research focusing on the subjective experiences of cancer patients undergoing somatic therapy, exploring themes like emotional well-being, coping mechanisms, and perceived benefits.

5. Comparative Studies: Papers that compare the effectiveness of somatic therapy with other forms of therapy or standard care in cancer treatment, looking at aspects like symptom management, emotional support, and overall health improvement.

6. Physiological Studies: Research exploring the biological or physiological changes associated with the practice of somatic therapies in cancer patients, such as changes in stress hormones, immune function, or pain perception.

7. Longitudinal Studies: Studies that follow cancer patients over time to assess the long-term effects of somatic therapy on health outcomes, recurrence rates, or survival.

8. Policy and Implementation Papers: Studies or reports discussing the integration of somatic therapies into standard cancer care, including challenges, guidelines, and recommendations for healthcare systems.

To find these papers, you can search academic databases such as PubMed, Google Scholar, JSTOR, and others. Using keywords like "somatic therapy," "cancer treatment," "mind-body therapies," "complementary therapies in oncology," and specific therapy types (e.g., "yoga," "mindfulness," "tai chi") in combination with "cancer" can help narrow down relevant research articles.

THE END